I0768055

STROKE:

30
POPULAR
FREQUENTLY ASKED QUESTIONS

1st Edition

Copyright © 2024 Hafifi Hisham All rights reserved

The characters and events portrayed in this book are fictitious. Any similarity to real persons, living or dead, is coincidental and not intended by the author.

No part of this book may be reproduced, stored in a retrieval system, or transmitted in any form or by any means, electronic, mechanical, photocopying, recording, or otherwise, without express written permission of the publisher.

NOOR HAFIFI NOORHISHAM

PHYSIOTHERAPY PROGRAM, CENTER FOR REHABILITATION AND SPECIAL NEEDS STUDIES, FACULTY OF HEALTH SCIENCES, UNIVERSITI KEBANGSAAN MALAYSIA, 50300 KUALA LUMPUR, MALAYSIA

ISBN: 979888327258425

February 2024

Cover design by: Art Painter

Library of Congress Control Number: 2018675309

Printed in the United States

EPIGRAPH

"In the journey through stroke, knowledge is the compass, resilience is the guide, and hope is the destination. This book is a lantern in the darkness, illuminating the path toward understanding, recovery, and renewed possibilities. As we explore the intricate tapestry of stroke together, may these pages inspire empowerment, foster compassion, and stand as a testament to the strength of the human spirit in the face of life-altering challenges."

— Anonymous

FOREWORD

In the face of a stroke, lives are abruptly rerouted, and the journey ahead often unfolds as uncharted territory, demanding resilience, understanding, and unwavering support. This book, ***"STROKE: 30 Popular Frequently Asked Questions"*** emerges as a beacon of knowledge and empathy, extending a compassionate hand to those navigating the aftermath of this life-altering event. As we embark on this exploration, the fusion of clinical expertise and personal narratives converges to create a resource that not only informs but also inspires. The voices within these pages are a testament to the indomitable human spirit, showcasing the strength and adaptability that define the stroke recovery journey.

From the foundational insights presented in the introduction to the nuanced responses provided in the frequently asked questions, this guide seeks to bridge the gap between medical understanding and the human experience. It is a collaborative effort, weaving together the threads of research, clinical practice, and the lived experiences of survivors and caregivers. In traversing these pages, readers will find not only answers to common questions about stroke but also a holistic perspective that embraces the multifaceted dimensions of recovery.

This foreword serves as an invitation to delve into a resource designed to inform, empower, and uplift—offering solace and understanding to those grappling with the complexities of stroke. May this guide illuminate the path forward, fostering a community bound by knowledge, compassion, and shared humanity.

— [Hafifi Hisham, PhD]

PROLOGUE

In the labyrinth of healthcare challenges, stroke stands as a formidable force, reshaping lives and testing the limits of resilience. This book emerges as a companion in the uncharted territory of stroke, offering a tapestry woven with threads of knowledge, experience, and hope. As we embark on this exploration, the echoes of countless narratives—of survivors, caregivers, and healthcare professionals—reverberate through these pages.

Within these words, we confront the complexities of stroke, unravel its mysteries, and navigate the winding paths of recovery. From the poignant stories of those who have faced this formidable adversary to the expertise of healthcare professionals steering the way, this prologue serves as an invitation to an odyssey of understanding, empathy, and empowerment.

PREFACE

Navigating the complexities of stroke and its aftermath can be a challenging journey. In this concise guide, we present answers to 30 popular questions about stroke, drawing from the expertise of healthcare professionals and the experiences of those who have traversed the path of recovery.

From understanding the signs and rehabilitation strategies to exploring lifestyle changes and support systems, this resource aims to empower individuals, caregivers, and the community at large. With a focus on clarity and accessibility, these insights offer valuable perspectives on stroke, fostering awareness, resilience, and a pathway to informed decision-making in the face of this life-altering event.

AUTHOR

Dr Noor Hafifi Noorhisham is a distinguished lecturer and researcher hailing from Universiti Kebangsaan Malaysia (Malaysian National University). With a robust academic background, he earned her PhD in Physiotherapy from Universiti Teknologi MARA (UiTM), Malaysia, showcasing a dedication to advancing knowledge in the field. Complementing his doctoral degree, he holds a Master's in Health Sciences and a Bachelor's (Hons) in Physiotherapy, both also from UiTM.

Dr Noor Hafifi brings a wealth of clinical experience to his academic role, boasting over a decade of expertise in neurorehabilitation as a clinical physiotherapist. His commitment to the field is further demonstrated by his previous services as a physiotherapist and branch manager at the Social Security Rehabilitation Centre in Malaysia. This hands-on experience not only enriches his academic endeavours but also positions him as a valuable contributor to the practical understanding of physiotherapy and neurorehabilitation.

His multidimensional background, encompassing academic achievements and extensive clinical involvement, underscores Dr. Noor Hafifi's commitment to advancing healthcare and rehabilitation practices in Malaysia and globally. As a lecturer and researcher, he continues to play a vital role in shaping the future of physiotherapy and contributing to the well-being of individuals through his expertise and dedication.

ACKNOWLEDGMENT

As I reflect on the creation of this book, I am deeply grateful for the unwavering support and inspiration that has fueled its development. To my late mother, Pauziah Md Basir, whose resilience and strength echo in the words on these pages—your spirit lives on in this endeavour.

To my beloved wife, Nasiha Shakina Shariffuddin, and our children, your understanding, patience, and encouragement have been the pillars of my journey. Your love has motivated me to explore the intricacies of stroke with compassion and dedication.

This book is a testament to the profound impact of family and loved ones in shaping the narrative of stroke, resilience, and hope.

TABLE OF CONTENT

CHAPTER FOUR

CHAPTER ONE

INTRODUCTION

Stroke, a sudden disruption of blood supply to the brain, is a profound and often life-altering event that transcends medical boundaries. In this exploration of stroke, we delve into the intricate web of its consequences, challenges, and the remarkable journey of recovery. Affecting millions worldwide, stroke unveils its complexity through the lens of physiology, rehabilitation, and the human spirit.

This comprehensive guide endeavours to demystify the enigma of stroke by addressing 30 frequently asked questions and providing insights into its causes, signs, and multifaceted recovery strategies. From understanding the vital importance of timely intervention to embracing the nuances of rehabilitation, we navigate the intricate landscape of stroke with empathy and expertise.

As we embark on this journey together, let us unravel the mysteries, confront the uncertainties, and celebrate the triumphs that define the post-stroke narrative. In the pursuit of knowledge, empowerment, and solidarity, this exploration seeks to not only inform but also inspire, offering a beacon of understanding for individuals, caregivers, and communities impacted by the profound

ripple effects of stroke.

CHAPTER TWO

30 POPULAR

FREQUENTLY ASKED QUESTIONS ON STROKE

1. WHAT IS A STROKE, AND HOW DOES IT AFFECT THE BODY?

A stroke occurs when the blood supply to a part of the brain is interrupted or reduced, leading to damage or death of brain cells (Andrabi et al., 2020; Orellana-Urzúa et al., 2020). This interruption can result from a blood clot blocking an artery (ischemic stroke) or a blood vessel bursting (haemorrhagic stroke) (Ye et al., 2021). The effects of a stroke depend on the area of the brain affected and the extent of damage (Murphy & Werring, 2020). Common consequences include paralysis or weakness on one side of the body, difficulty speaking or understanding language, and challenges with memory and cognitive functions. Quick medical intervention is crucial to minimize lasting effects and improve the chances of recovery (Kuriakose & Xiao, 2020).

2. WHY IS REHABILITATION IMPORTANT AFTER A STROKE?

Rehabilitation after a stroke is crucial for several reasons. Firstly, it helps individuals regain lost abilities, such as mobility, speech, and cognitive function, promoting independence in daily life (Murphy & Werring, 2020). Secondly, rehabilitation can prevent complications associated with immobility, such as muscle atrophy and joint stiffness (McGlinchey et al., 2020). Additionally, it addresses emotional and psychological aspects, aiding in coping with the changes brought about by a stroke (Smith et al., 2021). Rehabilitation maximizes the potential for recovery and enhances the overall quality of life (Teasell et al., 2020). Through targeted therapies and support, stroke survivors can optimize their physical and mental well-being, adapting to a new normal and achieving the highest level of functionality possible.

3. HOW SOON SHOULD STROKE REHABILITATION BEGIN?

Stroke rehabilitation ideally begins as soon as the individual is medically stable (Arsenault et al., 2024). In many cases, rehabilitation can commence within a few days after the stroke.

Early initiation of rehabilitation is crucial because the brain has a degree of plasticity, allowing it to reorganize and adapt (Aderinto et al., 2023). Starting rehabilitation promptly takes advantage of this neuroplasticity, enhancing the chances of recovery and minimizing potential complications (Liu et al., 2022). The specific timing may vary based on the individual's overall health, the severity of the stroke, and the recommendations of the medical team. However, the sooner rehabilitation begins, the better the outcomes in terms of functional improvement and recovery.

4. WHAT ARE THE COMMON SIGNS OF STROKE RECOVERY PROGRESS?

Common signs of stroke recovery progress include:

- **Improved Motor Skills:** Gradual regaining of strength and coordination, leading to increased control over movements.

- **Enhanced Speech and Communication:** Progress in speech therapy may result in improved articulation, fluency, and language comprehension.

- **Increased Independence in Activities of Daily Living (ADLs):** The ability to perform daily tasks independently, such as dressing, grooming, and eating.

- **Cognitive Improvement:** Advancements in memory, problem-solving, and other cognitive functions through rehabilitation efforts.

- **Reduced Dependence on Assistive Devices:** The need for mobility aids or assistive devices may decrease as physical function improves.

- **Emotional Well-Being:** Positive changes in mood and mental health, often aided by psychological support during rehabilitation.

- **Regained Sensation:** Recovery of sensory functions, such as touch and spatial awareness.

- **Adaptation to Lifestyle Changes:** Successful integration of lifestyle modifications is recommended for long-term stroke recovery.

Monitoring these signs helps healthcare professionals and individuals track progress, adjusting rehabilitation plans accordingly. It's essential to recognize and celebrate even small victories on the road to recovery.

5. CAN EVERYONE BENEFIT FROM STROKE REHABILITATION?

While the extent of benefit may vary, the majority of individuals who have experienced a stroke can benefit significantly from stroke rehabilitation. Rehabilitation is designed to address a range of challenges and deficits resulting from a stroke, including physical, cognitive, and emotional aspects. It aims to maximize one's functional abilities, enhance independence, and improve overall quality of life (McGlinchey et al., 2020). The specific benefits depend on factors such as the severity of the stroke, the individual's overall health, and the timely initiation of rehabilitation (Yochelson et al., 2021). Therefore, while not everyone's experience will be the same, stroke rehabilitation offers valuable support for most individuals on their journey to recovery.

6. WHAT ARE THE DIFFERENT TYPES OF STROKE REHABILITATION THERAPIES?

Stroke rehabilitation encompasses various therapies tailored to address specific aspects of recovery (Richards & Cramer, 2023). Common types include:

- **Physical Therapy (PT):** Focuses on improving mobility, balance, and coordination through targeted exercises and activities.

- **Occupational Therapy (OT):** Aim to enhance independence in daily activities, such as dressing, cooking, and personal care, by improving fine motor skills.

- **Speech-Language Therapy (SLT):** Addresses speech and communication challenges, as well as difficulties with swallowing.

- **Cognitive Therapy:** Targets cognitive functions like memory, problem-solving, and attention to improve overall cognitive abilities.

- **Recreational Therapy:** Uses leisure activities and exercises to enhance physical and mental well-being.

- **Aquatic Therapy:** Utilizes water exercises to improve strength, flexibility, and balance with reduced impact.

- **Constraint-Induced Movement Therapy (CIMT):** Restricts the use of the unaffected limb to encourage the use and improvement of the affected limb.

- **Music Therapy:** Utilizes music to address emotional and physical challenges, promoting relaxation and engagement.

- **Art Therapy:** Integrates creative expression to enhance emotional well-being and cognitive function.

- **Robotic-Assisted Therapy:** Involves the use of robotic devices to aid in repetitive, controlled movements for motor skill improvement.

- **Virtual Reality (VR) Therapy:** Uses simulated environments to engage patients in interactive activities, promoting motor and cognitive recovery.

The combination of these therapies is often tailored to an individual's specific needs, ensuring a comprehensive and personalized approach to stroke rehabilitation.

7. HOW LONG DOES A TYPICAL STROKE REHABILITATION SESSION LAST?

The duration of a stroke rehabilitation session can vary based on individual needs, the specific therapy involved, and the recommendations of the healthcare team. Typically, sessions range from 30 minutes to an hour, but this can be shorter or longer depending on factors such as the patient's tolerance, energy levels, and the intensity of the rehabilitation exercises. Additionally, some individuals may have multiple therapy sessions in a day, while others may have sessions spread throughout the week. The frequency and duration of sessions are often adjusted over time based on the individual's progress and rehabilitation goals.

8. ARE THERE HOME-BASED REHABILITATION OPTIONS FOR STROKE SURVIVORS?

Yes, home-based rehabilitation options are available and can be beneficial for stroke survivors. Home-based programs offer the flexibility to continue rehabilitation in a familiar environment (Chen et al., 2020). Here are some common home-based rehabilitation options:

- **Home Exercise Programs:** Tailored exercises designed to improve strength, flexibility, and mobility.

- **Daily Living Skills Training:** Practicing and enhancing activities of daily living (ADLs) such as dressing, grooming, and cooking.

- **Telehealth Sessions:** Virtual rehabilitation sessions with therapists via video calls for guidance and support.

- **Assistive Devices:** Using devices at home to aid mobility and independence, such as handrails, shower chairs, or adaptive utensils.

- **Cognitive Exercises:** Engaging in mental exercises to improve memory, attention, and problem-solving.

- **Adaptive Strategies:** Implementing strategies to overcome specific challenges in the home environment.

Home-based rehabilitation is often complemented by periodic visits to healthcare professionals for assessments and adjustments to the rehabilitation plan. It provides stroke survivors with ongoing support and promotes continuity in their recovery journey.

9. WHAT ROLE DOES PHYSICAL THERAPY (PT) PLAY IN STROKE REHABILITATION?

Physical Therapy (PT) plays a crucial role in stroke rehabilitation, addressing physical challenges and promoting overall recovery. Key aspects of the role of physical therapy in stroke rehabilitation include:

- **Mobility Improvement:** PT focuses on enhancing mobility, balance, and coordination, helping stroke survivors regain the ability to walk and move with greater confidence.

- **Strength Training:** Targeted exercises aim to rebuild strength in affected limbs, promoting muscle tone and reducing weakness.

- **Range of Motion Exercises:** PT helps restore flexibility and joint mobility, minimizing stiffness and preventing contractures.

- **Gait Training:** Rehabilitation includes techniques to improve walking patterns and reduce the risk of falls.

- **Functional Independence:** PT works towards improving the ability to perform daily activities independently, such as getting in and out of bed or navigating stairs.

- **Pain Management:** PT interventions may include strategies to alleviate pain associated with muscle tightness or joint stiffness.

- **Assistive Device Training:** Stroke survivors are taught how to use mobility aids such as canes, walkers, or braces to enhance stability.

- **Adaptation to Challenges:** Physical therapists help individuals adapt to challenges posed by weakness, spasticity, or sensory deficits.

- **Education and Home Exercise Programs:** PT provides guidance on home exercises and educates both the individual and their caregivers on maintaining progress outside of therapy sessions.

The goal of physical therapy in stroke rehabilitation is to optimize physical function, promote independence, and enhance the individual's overall quality of life (McGlinchey et al., 2020). The specific interventions are tailored to the unique needs and goals of each stroke survivor.

10. HOW DOES OCCUPATIONAL THERAPY (OT) HELP IN STROKE RECOVERY?

Occupational Therapy (OT) is integral to stroke recovery, focusing on enhancing the ability to perform daily activities and promoting independence. Here are key ways in which occupational therapy aids in stroke recovery:

- **Activities of Daily Living (ADL) Training:** OT addresses tasks like dressing, grooming, bathing, and cooking, helping individuals regain the skills necessary for self-care.

- **Fine Motor Skills Improvement:** Rehabilitation includes exercises to enhance hand-eye coordination, grip strength, and dexterity, enabling better control of small movements.

- **Cognitive Rehabilitation:** OT interventions target cognitive functions related to daily activities, such as memory, attention, and problem-solving.

- **Adaptive Techniques:** Occupational therapists introduce adaptive strategies and assistive devices to compensate for physical or cognitive challenges.

- **Home and Environmental Modifications:** OT assesses the home environment and recommends modifications to improve safety and accessibility.

- **Workplace Reintegration:** For those returning to work, OT assists in developing strategies to resume employment responsibilities effectively.

- **Sensory Integration:** Therapists address sensory deficits, working to improve sensory processing and enhance awareness of the surrounding environment.

- **Community Integration:** OT supports individuals in participating in social and community activities, fostering a sense of normalcy and inclusion.

- **Visual Perception Training:** Rehabilitation helps improve visual processing skills, aiding in tasks like reading, writing, and navigating the environment.

- **Psychosocial Support:** Occupational therapists address emotional well-being, providing support and strategies to cope with the psychological impact of stroke.

By addressing the practical challenges of daily life, occupational therapy plays a vital role in restoring a stroke survivor's functional independence and overall quality of life. The interventions are personalized to each individual's specific needs and goals.

11. IS SPEECH THERAPY IMPORTANT FOR ALL STROKE SURVIVORS?

Speech therapy, also known as speech-language therapy (SLT), is important for many stroke survivors, especially those who experience difficulties with speech, language, and swallowing. The need for speech therapy depends on the specific impact of the stroke on an individual. Here's why speech therapy is essential:

- **Speech and Articulation:** Speech therapy helps individuals improve their ability to speak clearly, addressing challenges with articulation and pronunciation.

- **Language Comprehension and Expression:** For those who have difficulty understanding or expressing language, speech therapy focuses on improving both receptive and expressive language skills.

- **Cognitive-Communication Skills:** Speech therapists work on enhancing cognitive-communication functions, such as memory, attention, and problem-solving related to communication.

- **Swallowing Rehabilitation:** Many stroke survivors experience dysphagia (difficulty swallowing), and speech therapy plays a key role in retraining swallowing muscles and improving safety during eating and drinking.

- **Voice Rehabilitation:** For those with changes in voice quality post-stroke, speech therapy can help restore and strengthen the voice.

- **Social Communication Skills:** Speech therapists address pragmatic language skills, helping individuals navigate social interactions and communication etiquette.

- **Alternative Communication Methods:** In cases where speech is severely affected, speech therapists may introduce alternative communication methods, such as communication devices or sign language.

While not all stroke survivors may require speech therapy, it is crucial for those facing challenges in these areas. The therapy is personalized to address the specific communication and swallowing needs of each individual, improving their overall quality of life and facilitating a smoother reintegration into daily activities.

12. WHAT DIETARY CONSIDERATIONS ARE CRUCIAL FOR STROKE RECOVERY?

Diet plays a crucial role in stroke recovery, contributing to overall health and well-being (Zielińska-Nowak et al., 2021). Here are key dietary considerations for stroke recovery:

- **Balanced Diet:** Emphasize a well-balanced diet rich in fruits, vegetables, whole grains, lean proteins, and healthy fats.

- **Hydration:** Maintain adequate hydration, as dehydration can exacerbate stroke-related complications.

- **Limit Sodium Intake:** Reduce sodium intake to help manage blood pressure, a critical factor in stroke prevention and recovery.

- **Heart-Healthy Fats:** Choose sources of healthy fats, such as avocados, nuts, seeds, and olive oil, to support cardiovascular health.

- **Omega-3 Fatty Acids:** Include fatty fish (salmon, mackerel) and flaxseeds for their anti-inflammatory and heart-protective properties.

- **Limit Saturated and Trans Fats:** Minimize intake of saturated and trans fats, found in processed foods and certain cooking oils.

- **Fibre-rich foods:** Opt for high-fibre foods to support digestive health and regulate cholesterol levels.

- **Control Blood Sugar Levels:** Monitor and manage blood sugar levels, especially for individuals with diabetes, as uncontrolled diabetes can complicate stroke recovery.

- **Calcium and Vitamin D:** Include sources of calcium and vitamin D for bone health, especially if there are mobility challenges.

- **Limit Added Sugars:** Minimize the intake of foods and beverages high in added sugars, as they can contribute to inflammation and weight gain.

- **Regular, Small Meals:** Consume regular, smaller meals to maintain energy levels and support metabolism.

Individual dietary needs may vary, and consultation with a healthcare professional or a registered dietitian is recommended to tailor dietary recommendations to the specific needs and health status of the individual. A healthy and nutrient-rich diet can contribute significantly to the recovery process after a stroke (Muscaritoli, 2021).

13. CAN TECHNOLOGY AID IN STROKE REHABILITATION?

Yes, technology can play a significant role in stroke rehabilitation, offering innovative solutions to enhance recovery (Kim et al., 2020). Here are ways in which technology aids in stroke rehabilitation:

- **Virtual Reality (VR) Therapy:** VR technology provides immersive environments for therapeutic exercises, improving motor skills, and spatial awareness.

- **Robot-Assisted Therapy:** Robotic devices assist in repetitive, controlled movements, promoting motor recovery and strength.

- **Wearable Devices:** Fitness trackers and smartwatches can monitor activity levels, encouraging individuals to stay active and providing valuable data for rehabilitation progress.

- **Telehealth Services:** Remote consultations and virtual therapy sessions allow individuals to receive ongoing support and guidance from healthcare professionals, especially useful for those with limited mobility.

- **Brain-Computer Interface (BCI):** BCI technology enables direct communication between the brain and external devices, potentially aiding in rehabilitation by controlling assistive devices.

- **Mobile Apps:** Numerous apps are designed for stroke survivors, offering exercises, cognitive games, and tools to track progress.

- **Adaptive Gaming:** Interactive games and gaming consoles with motion-sensing capabilities can make rehabilitation exercises more engaging.

- **Assistive Devices:** Various technological aids, such as voice-activated assistants and smart home devices, can enhance independence for stroke survivors with mobility or communication challenges.

- **Biofeedback Systems:** These systems provide real-time information on physiological processes, helping individuals gain awareness and control over certain functions, such as muscle activity.

- **Sensor Technology:** Wearable sensors can monitor movement patterns, providing valuable data for therapists to customize rehabilitation programs.

- **Functional Electrical Stimulation (FES):** FES devices use electrical currents to stimulate paralyzed or weakened muscles, aiding in functional movements.

The integration of technology into stroke rehabilitation not only makes therapy more engaging but also allows for more personalized and data-driven approaches, potentially accelerating the recovery process (Nizamis et al., 2021). However, these technologies need to be used under the guidance of healthcare professionals to ensure their appropriateness for individual needs.

14. WHAT IS NEUROPLASTICITY, AND HOW DOES IT RELATE TO STROKE REHABILITATION?

Neuroplasticity refers to the brain's ability to reorganize itself by forming new neural connections throughout life (Alia et al., 2017). It involves the brain's capacity to adapt and change in response to experiences, learning, and recovery from injury (Alia et al., 2017). This concept is particularly relevant in stroke rehabilitation.

When a stroke occurs, the brain's blood supply is disrupted, leading to the death of certain brain cells. Neuroplasticity allows the remaining healthy neurons to compensate for the lost functions by creating new connections and rerouting signals (Zotey et al., 2023). This process enables the brain to adapt to the damage caused by a stroke.

In the context of stroke rehabilitation, understanding and leveraging neuroplasticity are crucial. Rehabilitation exercises and therapies are designed to stimulate and reinforce specific neural pathways, encouraging the brain to reorganize and optimize its functioning (Su & Xu, 2020). Through targeted and repetitive activities, stroke survivors can promote the development of new neural connections, leading to improved motor skills, cognitive abilities, and overall recovery (Xing & Bai, 2020).

The principles of neuroplasticity highlight the importance of early and consistent rehabilitation efforts, as the brain is more receptive to change in the initial stages of recovery (Xing & Bai, 2020). Rehabilitation programs that take advantage of neuroplasticity aim to enhance the brain's ability to adapt and maximize the potential for functional improvement after a stroke.

15. HOW DO EMOTIONAL FACTORS IMPACT STROKE REHABILITATION?

Emotional factors play a significant role in stroke rehabilitation, influencing both the individual's well-being and the overall recovery process (Smith et al., 2021). Here are ways in which emotional factors impact stroke rehabilitation:

- **Motivation and Engagement:** Positive emotions and a motivated mindset can enhance a person's commitment to rehabilitation exercises and therapies, promoting active participation and engagement in the recovery process (Swaffield et al., 2022).

- **Stress and Anxiety:** High levels of stress and anxiety can negatively impact recovery by affecting cognitive function, increasing muscle tension, and hindering the ability to focus on rehabilitation tasks.

- **Depression:** Depression is a common emotional challenge after a stroke and can impede rehabilitation progress. It may lead to decreased motivation, fatigue, and social withdrawal.

- **Self-Efficacy:** Believing in one's ability to achieve rehabilitation goals (self-efficacy) is crucial. High self-efficacy is associated with better adherence to therapy and improved outcomes.

- **Social Support:** Emotional well-being is often influenced by the support system. Positive social interactions and support from family and friends contribute to a more positive emotional state.

- **Coping Strategies:** Emotional resilience and effective coping strategies can enhance the ability to navigate the challenges of stroke recovery, fostering a more positive mindset.

- **Fear of Falling:** Fear of falling can be a significant emotional barrier, limiting a person's willingness to engage in mobility exercises. Addressing this fear is essential for promoting physical activity and rehabilitation.

- **Frustration and Patience:** The frustration that may arise from the slow pace of recovery requires emotional resilience. Patience is vital, as progress in stroke rehabilitation often takes time.

Healthcare professionals, including therapists and psychologists, often incorporate psychological support into stroke rehabilitation programs to address emotional factors. By fostering a positive emotional environment, individuals are better equipped to navigate the challenges of recovery, adhere to rehabilitation plans, and ultimately enhance their overall well-being.

16. WHAT IS THE ROLE OF FAMILY SUPPORT IN STROKE RECOVERY?

Family support plays a crucial role in stroke recovery, contributing to both the emotional well-being of the stroke survivor and the overall success of rehabilitation (Lobo et al., 2023; Szczepańska-Gieracha & Mazurek, 2020). Here are key aspects of the role of family support in stroke recovery:

- **Emotional Support:** Family members provide emotional reassurance, understanding, and encouragement, helping the stroke survivor cope with the challenges and emotional impact of the stroke.

- **Motivation and Encouragement:** Positive reinforcement from family members can significantly motivate the stroke survivor to actively engage in rehabilitation activities, fostering a sense of purpose and determination.

- **Assistance with Daily Activities:** Family support often involves helping with daily tasks such as dressing, grooming, meal preparation, and transportation, especially in the early stages of recovery.

- **Communication Assistance:** For individuals facing speech and communication challenges, family members play a vital role in facilitating effective communication and understanding the needs and preferences of the stroke survivor.

- **Facilitating Rehabilitation Exercises:** Family members can actively participate in rehabilitation exercises recommended by healthcare professionals, providing guidance and assistance in practising therapeutic activities.

- **Advocacy in Healthcare Settings:** Families serve as advocates for the stroke survivor, ensuring effective communication with healthcare providers, understanding treatment plans, and participating in care decisions.

- **Providing a Supportive Home Environment:** Creating a home environment that is safe, accessible, and conducive to recovery is crucial. Family members may make necessary modifications and accommodations to facilitate rehabilitation.

- **Offering Social Support:** Family support helps alleviate feelings of isolation by facilitating social interactions, engaging in recreational activities, and providing opportunities for the stroke survivor to remain connected with the community.

- **Assisting with Medication Management:** Family members can assist in managing medication schedules, ensuring that the stroke survivor adheres to prescribed medications for optimal recovery.

- **Education and Information:** Families play a role in understanding the impact of stroke and the specifics of rehabilitation. Educated family members can provide better support and contribute to informed decision-making.

The collaborative efforts of healthcare professionals and supportive family members create an environment conducive to effective stroke recovery. Family involvement is instrumental in promoting the physical, emotional, and social well-being of the stroke survivor throughout the rehabilitation journey.

17. ARE THERE SPECIFIC EXERCISES FOR STROKE SURVIVORS TO DO AT HOME?

Yes, there are several home-based exercises that stroke survivors can do to complement their rehabilitation and promote ongoing recovery. However, individuals must consult with their healthcare team before starting any new exercise routine. Here are some general exercises that may be recommended for stroke survivors at home:

- **Range of Motion Exercises:**
  - Gently move each joint through its full range of motion to improve flexibility.

- **Strength Training:**

- o Use resistance bands or light weights for exercises targeting major muscle groups.

- **Balance Exercises:**

- o Stand near a sturdy surface and practice weight shifting, single-leg stands, and heel-to-toe walking.

- **Walking Exercises:**

- o Practice walking with proper posture and a steady gait, incorporating short walks into the daily routine.

- **Seated Exercises:**

- o Engage in seated exercises, such as leg lifts, seated marches, and seated leg extensions.

- **Hand and Finger Exercises:**

- o Practice fine motor exercises like picking up small objects, finger tapping, and hand squeezes.

- **Cognitive Exercises:**

- o Engage in activities that stimulate cognitive function, such as puzzles, memory games, and reading.

- **Stretching Exercises:**

- o Perform gentle stretches to improve flexibility and reduce muscle tightness.

- **Breathing Exercises:**

- o Practice deep breathing exercises to enhance lung capacity and relaxation.

- **Adaptive Yoga or Tai Chi:**

  - o Participate in adaptive yoga or Tai Chi programs designed for individuals with varying mobility levels.

Remember, the intensity and type of exercises should be tailored to the individual's abilities and limitations. Regular, consistent practice is essential for optimal results. It's advisable to work with a healthcare professional or a qualified therapist to create a personalized home exercise program that aligns with the individual's rehabilitation goals and overall health status.

18. CAN STROKE REHABILITATION IMPROVE MEMORY AND COGNITIVE FUNCTION?

Yes, stroke rehabilitation can contribute to improvements in memory and cognitive function (Lobo et al., 2023). Cognitive deficits, including memory challenges, are common after a stroke due to the disruption of blood flow and damage to brain cells. Here's how stroke rehabilitation can aid in enhancing memory and cognitive abilities:

- **Cognitive Therapy:** Specialized cognitive rehabilitation programs target specific cognitive functions, including memory. These may involve memory exercises, problem-solving tasks, and activities to improve attention and concentration.

- **Neuropsychological Interventions:** Neuropsychologists work with stroke survivors to assess cognitive strengths and weaknesses, developing interventions to address specific cognitive deficits.

- **Memory Training:** Therapists may employ memory training exercises, such as mnemonic strategies, repetition, and association techniques, to enhance memory recall.

- **Adaptive Strategies:** Rehabilitation focuses on teaching adaptive strategies to compensate for memory difficulties, enabling individuals to navigate daily tasks more effectively.

- **Technology-Assisted Cognitive Training:** Computer-based programs and apps designed for cognitive training can be incorporated into rehabilitation, providing interactive exercises to stimulate memory and cognitive function.

- **Functional Tasks Practice:** Engaging in real-world tasks during rehabilitation helps reinforce cognitive skills necessary for everyday activities, contributing to memory improvement.

- **Speech-Language Therapy:** Speech therapists address communication challenges, including those related to memory, by employing strategies to enhance language processing and expression.

- **Physical Exercise:** Regular physical activity has been linked to cognitive benefits. Exercise promotes blood flow to the brain, neuroplasticity, and the release of neuroprotective factors.

- **Lifestyle Modifications:** Addressing modifiable risk factors such as hypertension, and diabetes, and adopting a healthy lifestyle can contribute to overall cognitive health.

While rehabilitation can positively impact memory and cognitive function, the extent of improvement varies among individuals. The timing of rehabilitation initiation, the severity of the stroke, and the consistency of therapeutic interventions all play crucial roles in determining outcomes. A multidisciplinary approach involving occupational therapists, speech therapists, neuropsychologists, and other healthcare professionals is often key to addressing cognitive challenges comprehensively.

19. HOW LONG DOES IT TAKE TO REGAIN LOST MOTOR SKILLS AFTER A STROKE?

The timeline for regaining lost motor skills after a stroke varies widely among individuals and depends on several factors, including the severity of the stroke, the specific areas of the brain affected, the timeliness of rehabilitation, and the overall health of the individual (Clark et al., 2021). Recovery is a gradual process, and improvements may continue for months or even years after the initial stroke. Here are some general guidelines:

- **Early Recovery (Days to Weeks):** In the initial days and weeks after a stroke, individuals may experience spontaneous recovery, with some improvement in motor skills (Christian Grefkes & Gereon R Fink, 2020). Early rehabilitation efforts often focus on preventing complications and initiating basic movements.

- **Subacute Phase (Weeks to Months):** Substantial gains in motor skills often occur during the subacute phase, typically spanning several weeks to a few months (Koroleva et al., 2021). Intensive rehabilitation during this period is crucial, and individuals may achieve significant improvements in strength, coordination, and mobility (Christian Grefkes & Gereon R Fink, 2020).

- **Chronic Phase (Months to Years):** Recovery can continue over an extended period, with individuals making more gradual progress in refining and optimizing motor skills (Koroleva et al., 2021). Continued rehabilitation efforts may focus on fine-tuning movements, promoting independence, and addressing any persistent challenges (Christian Grefkes & Gereon R Fink, 2020).

- **Plateaus and Continued Progress:** Some individuals may experience plateaus in their recovery, where progress appears to slow down (Koroleva et al., 2021). However, ongoing rehabilitation, adaptive strategies, and a positive mindset can contribute to continued improvement over an extended period (Christian Grefkes & Gereon R Fink, 2020).

It's essential to recognize that the extent of recovery varies, and some individuals may not fully regain all lost motor skills. The goal of stroke rehabilitation is to maximize functional independence and enhance the overall quality of life. Rehabilitation programs are tailored to individual needs, and progress is monitored and adjusted accordingly. Early and consistent rehabilitation, along with a supportive environment and a positive attitude, can significantly impact the recovery trajectory.

20. ARE THERE SPECIALIZED REHABILITATION PROGRAMS FOR DIFFERENT TYPES OF STROKES?

Yes, there are specialized rehabilitation programs designed to address the unique challenges associated with different types of strokes. Rehabilitation plans are often tailored based on the specific characteristics of the stroke, including whether it is ischemic or haemorrhagic, the affected areas of the brain, and the resulting impairments. Here are some considerations for specialized stroke rehabilitation programs:

- **Ischemic Stroke Rehabilitation:**
  - Rehabilitation focuses on restoring blood flow and minimizing damage caused by the blood clot (Premilovac & Sutherland, 2023).
  - Physical therapy addresses motor deficits and mobility challenges resulting from the ischemic event.
  - Occupational therapy targets daily living activities, and speech therapy may be included if there are communication or cognitive issues.

- **Haemorrhagic Stroke Rehabilitation:**

  o Rehabilitation aims to manage bleeding, reduce pressure on the brain, and address complications associated with the haemorrhage (Premilovac & Sutherland, 2023).

  o Interventions may include monitoring and controlling blood pressure, minimizing risk factors, and preventing re-bleeding.

  o Physical, occupational, and speech therapies are tailored to address specific impairments resulting from haemorrhagic stroke.

- **Brainstem Stroke Rehabilitation:**

  o Brainstem strokes present unique challenges due to the critical functions controlled by this region.

  o Rehabilitation may involve specialized therapies to address difficulties with balance, coordination, and sensory functions.

  o Speech therapy may be crucial for addressing issues with swallowing and speech.

- **Cerebellar Stroke Rehabilitation:**

- Cerebellar strokes affect coordination and balance (Robles et al., 2023).

  - Rehabilitation focuses on restoring motor coordination, balance, and posture.

    control.

  - Coordination exercises and balance training are emphasized in physical therapy.

- **Frontal Lobe Stroke Rehabilitation:**

  - Frontal lobe strokes may impact executive functions, personality, and emotional regulation (Stubberud et al., 2020).

  - Rehabilitation includes cognitive and behavioural interventions, addressing challenges in planning, decision-making, and emotional control.

- **Temporal Lobe Stroke Rehabilitation:**

  - Temporal lobe strokes may affect memory and auditory processing (Lwi et al., 2021).

Cognitive rehabilitation and memory training are important components, often involving speech and occupational therapy. Rehabilitation plans are highly individualized, considering the specific effects of the stroke on each person. The interdisciplinary approach involving physical therapists, occupational therapists, speech therapists, and other specialists ensures a comprehensive and personalized approach to stroke recovery.

21. WHAT IS THE IMPACT OF AGE ON STROKE REHABILITATION OUTCOMES?

Age can have an impact on stroke rehabilitation outcomes, influencing the rate and extent of recovery (Christian Grefkes & Gereon R. Fink, 2020). However, it's important to note that individuals of all ages can make significant progress with appropriate rehabilitation efforts. Here are some considerations regarding the impact of age on stroke rehabilitation outcomes:

- **Younger Age:**
    - Younger individuals may generally experience a faster rate of recovery due to potentially better overall health and resilience (Bartholomé & Winter, 2020).
    - They may be more likely to participate actively in rehabilitation programs, leading to improved outcomes.
    - Younger age may be associated with a greater capacity for neuroplasticity, allowing for more significant

reorganization and adaptation of the brain (Marzola et al., 2023).

- **Older Age:**
  - Older individuals may face additional challenges due to age-related factors such as pre-existing health conditions, reduced muscle mass, and decreased bone density (Purohit et al., 2023).
  - There may be a higher likelihood of comorbidities that could impact rehabilitation progress.
  - Older adults may experience a slower rate of recovery, and the extent of functional improvement may vary (Buvarp et al., 2020).

- **Individual Variability:**
  - While age is a factor, individual variability is substantial. Factors such as overall health, motivation, pre-stroke functional status, and the severity of the stroke play crucial roles (Christian Grefkes & Gereon R. Fink, 2020).
  - Some older individuals may exhibit remarkable resilience and make significant gains in rehabilitation (Smith et al., 2021).

- **Cognitive Impacts:**

o Age can influence cognitive reserve, with younger individuals potentially having greater cognitive reserve, allowing for better adaptation to brain changes (Yochelson et al., 2021).

o However, cognitive interventions and rehabilitation strategies can be effective across age groups.

- **Psychosocial Factors:**

o Psychosocial factors, including emotional well-being and social support, can influence rehabilitation outcomes in individuals of all ages (Stubberud et al., 2020).

- **Rehabilitation Approach:**

- The choice of rehabilitation approach may need to be tailored based on age-related considerations, such as incorporating activities that align with lifestyle preferences and functional goals.

It's crucial to approach stroke rehabilitation as an individualized process, considering the unique characteristics of each person. Rehabilitation plans should be adapted to the specific needs, goals, and capacities of the individual, regardless of age. The multidisciplinary healthcare team collaborates to create a personalized approach, optimizing outcomes for stroke survivors of all ages.

22. HOW CAN FATIGUE BE MANAGED DURING STROKE RECOVERY?

Fatigue is a common challenge during stroke recovery, impacting both physical and cognitive aspects of daily life (Lanctôt et al., 2020). Managing fatigue involves a combination of lifestyle adjustments, rehabilitation strategies, and self-care (Rahman et al., 2023). Here are some practical tips for managing fatigue during stroke recovery:

- **Prioritize Rest and Sleep:**
  - Ensure adequate and quality sleep by maintaining a consistent sleep schedule and creating a comfortable sleep environment.

- **Pacing Activities:**
  - Break down tasks into smaller, manageable segments, and take breaks between activities to prevent excessive exertion.

- **Energy Conservation:**

- Use energy-efficient strategies, such as sitting while performing tasks, using assistive devices, and optimizing the environment to minimize physical effort.

- **Set Realistic Goals:**

  - Establish achievable and realistic goals for daily activities, focusing on gradual progress rather than overwhelming tasks.

- **Balance Activity and Rest:**

  - Alternate periods of activity with periods of rest to prevent fatigue accumulation. This can involve short rest breaks during tasks.

- **Stay Hydrated:**

  - Maintain proper hydration levels, as dehydration can contribute to fatigue.

- **Nutrition:**

  - Consume a balanced diet to provide the necessary nutrients for energy. Consult a dietitian for personalized nutrition advice.

- **Manage Stress:**

- Practice stress-reducing techniques, such as deep breathing, meditation, or mindfulness, to manage emotional fatigue.

- **Exercise:**

  - Engage in appropriate and prescribed exercise programs to build stamina and strength gradually.

- **Adaptive Strategies:**

  - Use assistive devices or adaptive techniques to make activities less demanding, reducing the overall energy expenditure.

- **Evaluate Medications:**

  - Consult with healthcare professionals to review medications, as certain medications may contribute to fatigue.

- **Cognitive Rest:**

  - Incorporate breaks during cognitive activities, such as reading or using a computer, to prevent mental fatigue.

- **Simplify Tasks:**

  - Simplify tasks by breaking them into smaller steps, making them more manageable and less mentally taxing.

- **Rehabilitation Programs:**

  - Participate in tailored rehabilitation programs focusing on energy conservation techniques and gradual functional improvement.

- **Social Support:**

  - Seek support from family, friends, and healthcare professionals. Communicate your needs and limitations to avoid overexertion.

It's essential for individuals recovering from a stroke to communicate openly with their healthcare team about fatigue levels and to actively participate in developing strategies for managing fatigue. Adjustments to the rehabilitation plan and lifestyle modifications can be made to address individual needs and optimize recovery outcomes.

23. ARE THERE ALTERNATIVE THERAPIES FOR STROKE REHABILITATION?

Yes, several alternative therapies and complementary approaches may be considered as part of a holistic stroke rehabilitation plan. It's crucial to integrate these therapies under the guidance of healthcare professionals and in conjunction with conventional rehabilitation methods. Here are some alternative therapies that may be explored:

- **Acupuncture:**

  - Acupuncture involves the insertion of thin needles into specific points of the body to promote energy flow and balance. It may help with pain management, stress reduction, and overall well-being.

- **Massage Therapy:**

  - Massage can be beneficial for improving circulation, reducing muscle tension, and promoting relaxation. It may contribute to improved mobility and comfort.

- **Yoga:**

  - Adaptive or gentle yoga practices can help enhance flexibility, balance, and relaxation. Yoga may also contribute to stress reduction and emotional well-being.

- **Tai Chi:**

  - Tai Chi involves slow, flowing movements that can improve balance, coordination, and muscle strength. It is often considered a safe and low-impact exercise.

- **Art Therapy:**

- Engaging in artistic activities may provide a creative outlet for self-expression and emotional well-being. Art therapy can be adapted to address cognitive and motor challenges.

- **Music Therapy:**

  - Music therapy involves using music to address physical, emotional, and cognitive needs. It may help improve mood, reduce anxiety, and enhance cognitive function.

- **Aquatic Therapy:**

  - Exercising in water can reduce the impact on joints and muscles. Aquatic therapy may enhance mobility, strength, and balance.

- **Mind-Body Practices:**

  - Mindfulness, meditation, and guided imagery can contribute to stress reduction, relaxation, and improved focus. Mind-body practices may complement cognitive rehabilitation.

- **Animal-Assisted Therapy:**

  - Interacting with animals, such as therapy dogs, may provide emotional support and motivation during rehabilitation. This can contribute to increased social engagement.

- **Herbal and Dietary Supplements:**

  - Some individuals explore the use of herbal supplements or dietary changes under the guidance of healthcare professionals. It's essential to discuss these options with a healthcare provider to ensure safety and compatibility with medications.

- **Biofeedback:**

  - Biofeedback involves learning to control physiological processes, such as muscle tension or heart rate, using feedback from monitoring devices. It can be applied to various aspects of stroke rehabilitation.

Before incorporating alternative therapies, it's crucial to consult with healthcare professionals to ensure that these approaches align with the individual's specific needs, medical history, and rehabilitation goals. Integrative care, combining conventional and alternative therapies, can provide a more comprehensive and personalized approach to stroke recovery.

24. CAN STROKES CAUSE LONG-TERM DISABILITY, EVEN WITH REHABILITATION?

Yes, strokes can cause long-term disability, and the extent of disability can vary widely among individuals (Yochelson et al., 2021). Despite rehabilitation efforts, some stroke survivors may experience persistent impairments that significantly impact their daily functioning. The severity of the stroke, the specific areas of the brain affected, and the effectiveness of rehabilitation all play roles in determining the long-term outcomes.

Common long-term disabilities after a stroke may include:

- **Motor Impairments:**
  - Weakness or paralysis in one or more limbs, affecting mobility and coordination.
  - Challenges in balance and coordination, lead to an increased risk of falls.

- **Communication Difficulties:**
  - Aphasia, which can affect language comprehension, expression, reading, and writing.
  - Apraxia impacts the ability to carry out purposeful movements, such as speech or gestures.

- **Cognitive Challenges:**

- o Memory deficits, attention difficulties, and problems with executive functions (planning, decision-making).

  - o Challenges in problem-solving and multitasking.

- **Sensory Changes:**

  - o Changes in sensation, such as numbness or tingling in affected limbs.

  - o Visual impairments, including loss of vision or difficulty with visual processing.

- **Emotional and Psychological Impact:**

  - o Depression, anxiety, and emotional changes may persist, affecting overall well-being.

  - o Coping with the psychological impact of disability and adjusting to life changes.

It's important to note that rehabilitation can significantly improve functional outcomes and quality of life for many stroke survivors. Early and consistent rehabilitation efforts, along with a supportive environment, contribute to maximizing recovery potential (Christian Grefkes & Gereon R Fink, 2020). However, complete recovery is not always achievable, and some individuals may face long-term challenges.

The multidisciplinary rehabilitation team, including physical therapists, occupational therapists, speech therapists, and psychologists, collaborates to address the diverse needs of stroke survivors. The focus is on enhancing independence, promoting adaptive strategies, and improving overall quality of life. Regular follow-ups with healthcare professionals help monitor progress and make adjustments to rehabilitation plans as needed. Additionally, ongoing support from family and caregivers is crucial in facilitating long-term adaptation and coping with the challenges of stroke-related disabilities.

25. WHAT ASSISTIVE DEVICES ARE AVAILABLE TO AID IN STROKE RECOVERY?

Assistive devices play a valuable role in supporting stroke survivors during their recovery, helping them regain independence and perform daily activities. The selection of assistive devices depends on the specific challenges faced by the individual. Here are some common assistive devices used in stroke recovery:

- **Canes and Walkers:**
  - Canes provide stability and support for individuals with mild balance issues.

o Walkers offer increased support and stability for those with more significant mobility challenges.

- **Orthoses (Braces):**

  o Ankle-foot orthoses (AFOs) can assist with foot drop, helping control ankle movement and improving gait.

- **Wheelchairs and Mobility Scooters:**

  o Manual or powered wheelchairs can be used for mobility, especially if walking is challenging.

  o Mobility scooters provide an alternative for individuals with limited walking ability.

- **Transfer Aids:**

  o Transfer boards and transfer poles assist with moving between surfaces, such as from a bed to a chair.

- **Adaptive Utensils:**

  o Utensils with special grips or handles make eating easier for individuals with hand weakness or coordination issues.

- **Reacher/Grabber Tools:**

  o These tools help individuals reach objects on high shelves or pick up items from the floor without excessive bending.

- **Elevated Toilet Seats and Grab Bars:**

  o Modifications to the bathroom, such as elevated toilet seats and grab bars, enhance safety and independence.

- **Dressing Aids:**

  o Button hooks, zipper pulls, and dressing sticks assist with putting on and taking off clothing.

- **Adaptive Technology:**

  o Voice-activated devices, tablets, and smartphones with accessibility features can assist with communication, reminders, and daily tasks.

- **Communication Devices:**

  o Devices like speech-generating devices or communication apps can aid individuals with aphasia or communication difficulties.

- **Orthopedic Shoes and Insoles:**

  o Specialized footwear can help with foot stability and comfort, addressing issues related to gait and balance.

- **Adaptive Vehicle Modifications:**

  o Vehicle modifications, such as hand controls or wheelchair lifts, can enable individuals to drive or travel more independently.

- **Voice Recognition Software:**

  o Software that converts spoken words into text can assist with computer use for individuals with limited hand dexterity.

- **Stairlifts and Ramps:**

  o These modifications can enhance accessibility in homes with stairs, making it easier for individuals with mobility challenges.

Assistive devices are often prescribed or recommended by healthcare professionals as part of a comprehensive rehabilitation plan. Occupational therapists, physical therapists, and other specialists assess individual needs and guide on selecting and using appropriate assistive devices to improve functional abilities and promote independence.

26. HOW CAN CAREGIVERS SUPPORT STROKE SURVIVORS DURING REHABILITATION?

Caregivers play a crucial role in supporting stroke survivors during rehabilitation. Their involvement can significantly impact the overall well-being and recovery of the individual (Kokorelias et al., 2020). Here are ways caregivers can provide support during the rehabilitation process:

- **Attend Rehabilitation Sessions:**
  - Accompany the stroke survivor to rehabilitation sessions to gain an understanding of exercises and strategies to support ongoing progress at home.

- **Communication with the Healthcare Team:**
  - Maintain open communication with the healthcare team, including therapists and doctors, to stay informed about the individual's progress, goals, and any modifications to the rehabilitation plan.

- **Assist with Daily Activities:**
  - Help with daily activities, such as dressing, grooming, and preparing meals, as needed. Encourage independence while providing necessary support.

- **Encourage Mobility and Exercise:**
  - Support and encourage prescribed exercises and mobility activities. Ensure a safe environment for practising exercises and moving around the home.

- **Medication Management:**

- Assist with medication management, including organizing medications, reminding the individual to take them, and communicating with healthcare providers about any concerns.

- **Provide Emotional Support:**

  - Offer emotional support and encouragement. Be patient and understanding of the challenges the stroke survivor may be facing.

- **Encourage Social Engagement:**

  - Facilitate social interactions by organizing visits with friends and family or participating in group activities. Social engagement can contribute to emotional well-being.

- **Promote Independence:**

  - Encourage and support the stroke survivor in regaining independence. Focus on achievable goals and celebrate milestones along the way.

- **Address Safety Concerns:**

  - Assess the home environment for safety hazards and make necessary modifications. This includes

installing grab bars, removing tripping hazards, and
ensuring good lighting.

- **Educate Yourself:**

  o Learn about the effects of stroke, rehabilitation
  techniques, and any specific recommendations from
  healthcare professionals. Knowledge empowers
  caregivers to provide more effective support.

- **Advocate for the Stroke Survivor:**

  o Act as an advocate for stroke survivors in healthcare
  settings, ensuring that their needs and preferences are
  communicated effectively.

- **Seek Respite and Support:**

  o Caregivers should prioritize self-care and seek
  support when needed. Taking breaks and addressing
  their well-being contributes to their ability to provide
  effective care.

- **Adapt to Changing Needs:**

  o Be flexible and adapt to the changing needs of the
  stroke survivor. Rehabilitation goals and strategies
  may evolve, requiring adjustments in caregiving
  approaches.

- **Communication Assistance:**

  o Assist with communication, especially if the stroke survivor is experiencing speech or language difficulties. Use clear and simple language and encourage the use of communication aids if necessary.

Caregivers are essential partners in the rehabilitation journey, and their commitment and support significantly contribute to the success of the stroke survivor's recovery. Open communication, collaboration with healthcare professionals, and a compassionate approach are key elements in providing effective care.

27. ARE THERE COMMUNITY RESOURCES FOR STROKE SURVIVORS AFTER REHABILITATION?

Yes, there are various community resources and support services available for stroke survivors after rehabilitation. These resources aim to assist individuals in transitioning back into their communities, promoting ongoing recovery, and enhancing overall well-being (Magwood et al., 2020). Here are some common community resources for stroke survivors:

- **Stroke Support Groups:**

- o Local support groups provide a platform for stroke survivors to connect with others who have experienced similar challenges. These groups often offer emotional support, information sharing, and a sense of community.

- **Community Centres:**

  - o Many community centres offer programs and activities tailored for older adults and individuals with disabilities. These may include fitness classes, social events, and educational workshops.

- **Adaptive Recreation Programs:**

  - o Adaptive sports and recreation programs provide opportunities for individuals with mobility challenges to engage in physical activities, fostering social interaction and overall well-being.

- **Home Health Services:**

  - o Home health agencies offer services such as physical therapy, occupational therapy, and nursing care in the home environment, promoting continued recovery and independence.

- **Senior Centres:**

o Senior centres often provide a range of services, including social activities, health and wellness programs, and educational opportunities. These centres can be valuable for stroke survivors seeking community engagement.

- **Transportation Services:**

  o Accessible transportation services may be available to assist stroke survivors in getting to medical appointments, social activities, and other community events.

- **Meal Delivery Programs:**

  o Meal delivery services can provide nutritious meals for individuals who may face challenges with meal preparation.

- **Volunteer Services:**

  o Local volunteer organizations may offer assistance with various tasks, such as grocery shopping, transportation, or companionship.

- **Assistive Technology Centres:**

- o Centres specializing in assistive technology can help individuals explore and acquire devices that enhance independence, communication, and accessibility.

- **Educational Workshops:**

  - o Workshops on topics such as stroke prevention, healthy living, and managing post-stroke challenges may be available in the community.

- **Rehabilitation Centres and Clinics:**

  - o Outpatient rehabilitation centres provide ongoing therapy services, allowing stroke survivors to continue working on specific goals and maintaining functional gains.

- **Counselling and Mental Health Services:**

  - o Counselling services, including individual or family therapy, can address emotional challenges and support mental well-being.

- **Legal Aid Services:**

  - o Legal aid organizations may offer assistance with issues related to disability rights, insurance, and other legal matters.

- **Respite Care Services:**

- o Respite care services provide temporary relief for caregivers, allowing them to take breaks while ensuring the well-being of the stroke survivor.

Connecting with local healthcare providers, community organizations, and social services can help stroke survivors and their caregivers access available resources. Many communities have dedicated programs to support individuals in their post-rehabilitation journey, promoting a more inclusive and supportive environment.

28. WHAT IS CONSTRAINT-INDUCED MOVEMENT THERAPY, AND HOW EFFECTIVE IS IT?

Constraint-Induced Movement Therapy (CIMT) is a rehabilitation approach designed to improve the function of an affected limb after a stroke or other neurological injuries (Wang et al., 2022). The therapy involves restricting the use of the unaffected limb (usually the arm) while intensively training and encouraging the use of the affected limb (Abdullahi et al., 2021). The goal is to overcome learned non-use and promote neuroplasticity, the brain's ability to reorganize and adapt (Abdullahi et al., 2021).

Here's how CIMT typically works:

- **Constraint of the Unaffected Limb:**

  - The unaffected limb is constrained, often through the use of a mitt or sling, limiting its movement and forcing the individual to rely more on the affected limb.

- **Intensive Task-Specific Training:**

  - The individual engages in intensive and repetitive task-specific training using the affected limb. This involves practising functional activities that are relevant to daily life.

- **Shaping and Graded Tasks:**

  - Tasks are initially designed to be achievable but challenging. As the individual progresses, tasks become more complex and demanding, promoting motor skill development.

- **Behavioural Techniques:**

  - Behavioural techniques, including positive reinforcement and encouragement, are often incorporated to enhance motivation and engagement.

  - The effectiveness of CIMT has been studied extensively, and research suggests positive outcomes for certain populations. Key findings and considerations include:

- **Improved Arm Function:**
  - o CIMT has shown effectiveness in improving arm function, motor control, and coordination in individuals with mild to moderate upper limb impairment after stroke.

- **Enhanced Use of Affected Limb:**
  - o By encouraging and forcing increased use of the affected limb, CIMT aims to overcome learned non-use, where individuals avoid using the impaired limb due to initial difficulties.

- **Neuroplastic Changes:**
  - o CIMT is believed to induce neuroplastic changes in the brain, promoting the reorganization of neural pathways and enhancing recovery.

- **Best Suited for Specific Cases:**
  - o CIMT is often more effective for individuals with some residual movement in the affected limb, making it better suited for those with mild to moderate impairment.

- **Timing of Intervention:**

  o The timing of CIMT may influence its effectiveness. Early initiation of CIMT, typically within the first few months after a stroke, has shown positive results.

- **Individual Variability:**

  o Responses to CIMT can vary among individuals. Factors such as motivation, severity of impairment, and overall health may influence outcomes.

While CIMT has demonstrated positive effects in various studies, it may not be suitable or effective for everyone. The decision to use CIMT should be made in consultation with healthcare professionals who can assess the individual's specific needs and determine the most appropriate rehabilitation approach. The therapy is often part of a comprehensive rehabilitation plan tailored to the individual's goals and functional abilities.

29. CAN STROKE REHABILITATION IMPROVE BALANCE AND COORDINATION?

Yes, stroke rehabilitation can play a crucial role in improving balance and coordination for individuals who have experienced a stroke (Yu et al., 2021). Stroke often affects the brain's control over movement and balance, leading to deficits in these areas. Rehabilitation programs, including targeted exercises and therapies, are designed to address these deficits and promote recovery. Here's how stroke rehabilitation can help improve balance and coordination:

- **Physical Therapy:**
    - Physical therapists assess the individual's specific impairments and design exercises to improve strength, flexibility, and coordination. These exercises may target specific muscle groups involved in balance and gait.

- **Balance Training:**
    - Balance exercises are a key component of stroke rehabilitation. These exercises focus on improving postural control and stability. Common balance exercises include weight shifting, standing on one leg, and dynamic movements.

- **Gait Training:**
    - Gait training involves working on the individual's ability to walk. This may include exercises to improve step length, stride symmetry, and overall walking pattern.

Assistive devices like walkers or canes may be used as needed.

- **Coordination Exercises:**

  o Coordination exercises help improve the synchronization of movements. These may involve activities such as reaching, grasping objects, and hand-eye coordination exercises.

- **Functional Tasks Practice:**

  o Rehabilitation often includes practising functional tasks relevant to daily life. This may include activities like getting up from a chair, reaching for items on shelves, or navigating stairs.

- **Task-Specific Training:**

  o Task-specific training focuses on practising specific activities that challenge and improve coordination. For example, practising reaching and grasping objects of varying sizes and shapes.

- **Adaptive Techniques:**

  o Rehabilitation professionals teach adaptive techniques to compensate for specific balance and coordination deficits. This may include strategies for improving stability during transfers or using assistive devices.

- **Technology-Assisted Rehabilitation:**

  o Virtual reality and other technology-assisted rehabilitation methods can be used to provide engaging and targeted exercises for improving balance and coordination.

- **Aquatic Therapy:**

  o Aquatic therapy, conducted in a pool, can provide a buoyant environment that reduces the impact on joints while enhancing balance, strength, and coordination.

- **Feedback and Biofeedback:**

  o Real-time feedback during exercises, including visual or auditory cues, can help individuals make adjustments to improve balance and coordination.

The effectiveness of rehabilitation in improving balance and coordination can vary depending on the severity of the stroke, the individual's overall health, and the timing of intervention. Early and consistent rehabilitation efforts are generally associated with better outcomes. Rehabilitation programs are often tailored to the specific needs and goals of the individual, with ongoing assessment and adjustments as needed. The collaboration of physical therapists, occupational therapists, and other healthcare professionals is essential in addressing these aspects of recovery comprehensively.

30. WHAT LIFESTYLE CHANGES ARE RECOMMENDED FOR STROKE SURVIVORS POST-REHABILITATION?

After stroke rehabilitation, adopting certain lifestyle changes is crucial for promoting long-term health, preventing further strokes, and maintaining overall well-being (Stulberg et al., 2023). These changes often focus on risk factor management, healthy habits, and ongoing self-care. Here are recommended lifestyle changes for stroke survivors:

- **Medication Adherence:**
  - Take prescribed medications as directed by healthcare professionals. Medications may include blood thinners, antihypertensives, and cholesterol-lowering drugs to manage risk factors.

- **Regular Medical Check-ups:**
  - Attend regular follow-up appointments with healthcare providers to monitor blood pressure, cholesterol levels,

and overall health. These check-ups help detect and address potential issues early.

- **Healthy Diet:**

  o Adopt a heart-healthy diet that includes plenty of fruits, vegetables, whole grains, lean proteins, and low-fat dairy products. Limit sodium intake to support blood pressure control.

- **Regular Exercise:**

  o Engage in regular physical activity based on individual capabilities and recommendations from healthcare professionals. Exercise helps improve cardiovascular health, strength, and overall well-being.

- **Smoking Cessation:**

  o If the individual smokes, quitting is essential. Smoking is a significant risk factor for stroke and other cardiovascular diseases.

- **Moderate Alcohol Consumption:**

  o Limit alcohol intake to moderate levels or as recommended by healthcare providers. Excessive alcohol consumption can contribute to hypertension and other health issues.

- **Weight Management:**

o Maintain a healthy weight through a combination of a balanced diet and regular physical activity. Achieving and maintaining a healthy weight helps manage cardiovascular risk factors.

- **Stress Management:**

o Practice stress-reducing techniques such as deep breathing, meditation, yoga, or mindfulness. Managing stress contributes to overall cardiovascular health.

- **Regular Sleep:**

o Aim for adequate and quality sleep each night. Establishing a consistent sleep routine supports overall health and well-being.

- **Hydration:**

o Stay adequately hydrated by drinking plenty of water. Proper hydration is important for overall health and can contribute to optimal functioning.

- **Home Safety Measures:**

o Make home modifications to reduce the risk of falls. This may include installing grab bars, removing tripping hazards, and ensuring good lighting.

- **Social Engagement:**

- o Stay socially connected with friends, family, and community. Social engagement contributes to emotional well-being.

- **Cognitive Stimulation:**

  - o Engage in activities that stimulate the mind, such as reading, puzzles, and social interactions. Cognitive stimulation supports overall brain health.

- **Adaptive Strategies:**

  - o Continue using adaptive strategies learned during rehabilitation to address specific challenges. This may include the use of assistive devices or modified techniques for daily tasks.

- **Regular Dental Check-ups:**

  - o Schedule regular dental check-ups to maintain oral health. Periodontal disease has been linked to an increased risk of stroke.

Individuals should work closely with their healthcare team to develop a personalized plan that addresses their specific needs and risk factors. These lifestyle changes are not only beneficial for stroke survivors but are generally applicable to promoting cardiovascular health for the broader population.

CHAPTER FOUR

SUMMARY AND CONCLUSIONS

"STROKE: 30 Popular Frequently Asked Questions" is an illuminating book that addresses 30 pivotal questions surrounding the intricate landscape of stroke. Through a lens of compassion and expertise, this guide offers insights into the causes, signs, and multifaceted recovery strategies associated with stroke—a sudden and life-altering disruption of blood supply to the brain.

Navigating the complexities of stroke with clarity, the book covers crucial topics, including timely intervention, rehabilitation nuances, and the emotional dimensions of recovery. Drawing from the experiences of healthcare professionals, the narratives of survivors, and the collective wisdom of those who have confronted this medical challenge, the guide seeks to empower individuals, caregivers, and communities.

With a thoughtful preface acknowledging the impact of stroke and an introduction that sets the stage for understanding, this guide is a testament to resilience, hope, and the transformative power of knowledge. It stands as a beacon for those seeking to comprehend and navigate the challenges posed by stroke, fostering awareness, and offering practical insights that extend beyond medical boundaries. This comprehensive

resource invites readers on a journey of discovery, solidarity, and

empowerment in the face of one of life's profound health challenges.

REFERENCES

Abdullahi, A., Truijen, S., Umar, N. A., Useh, U., Egwuonwu, V. A., Van Criekinge, T., & Saeys, W. (2021). Effects of lower limb constraint induced movement therapy in people with stroke: A systematic review and meta-analysis. *Frontiers in neurology, 12*, 638904.

Aderinto, N., AbdulBasit, M. O., Olatunji, G., & Adejumo, T. (2023). Exploring the transformative influence of neuroplasticity on stroke rehabilitation: a narrative review of current evidence. *Annals of Medicine and Surgery, 85*(9). https://journals.lww.com/annals-of-medicine-and-surgery/fulltext/2023/09000/exploring_the_transformative_influence_of.38.aspx

Alia, C., Spalletti, C., Lai, S., Panarese, A., Lamola, G., Bertolucci, F., Vallone, F., Di Garbo, A., Chisari, C., & Micera, S. (2017). Neuroplastic changes following brain ischemia and their contribution to stroke recovery: novel approaches in neurorehabilitation. *Frontiers in cellular neuroscience, 11*, 76.

Andrabi, S. S., Parvez, S., & Tabassum, H. (2020). Ischemic stroke and mitochondria: mechanisms and targets. *Protoplasma, 257*(2), 335-343. https://doi.org/10.1007/s00709-019-01439-2

Arsenault, S., Bickford, D., Derbyshire, D., Doucette, S., Dowlatshahi, D., Foley, N., Ganesh, A., Ghrooda, E., Gubitz, G., Harris, D., Heran, M., Hill, M. D., Kanya-Forstner, N., Kaplovitch, E., Liederman, Z., Lindsay, P., Lund, R., Martin, C., Martiniuk, S., . . . van Adel, B. (2024). Canadian Stroke Best Practice Recommendations: Acute Stroke Management, 7th Edition Practice Guidelines Update, 2022. *Canadian Journal of Neurological Sciences / Journal Canadien des Sciences Neurologiques, 51*(1), 1-31. https://doi.org/10.1017/cjn.2022.344

Bartholomé, L., & Winter, Y. (2020). Quality of Life and Resilience of Patients With Juvenile Stroke: A Systematic Review. *Journal of Stroke and Cerebrovascular Diseases, 29*(10), 105129. https://doi.org/https://doi.org/10.1016/j.jstrokecerebrovasdis.2020.105129

Buvarp, D., Rafsten, L., & Sunnerhagen, K. S. (2020). Predicting Longitudinal Progression in Functional Mobility After Stroke. *Stroke, 51*(7), 2179-2187. https://doi.org/10.1161/STROKEAHA.120.029913

Chen, Y., Chen, Y., Zheng, K., Dodakian, L., See, J., Zhou, R., Chiu, N., Augsburger, R., McKenzie, A., & Cramer, S. C. (2020). A qualitative study on user acceptance of a home-based stroke telerehabilitation system. *Topics in Stroke Rehabilitation, 27*(2), 81-92. https://doi.org/10.1080/10749357.2019.1683792

Clark, B., Whitall, J., Kwakkel, G., Mehrholz, J., Ewings, S., & Burridge, J. (2021). The effect of time spent in rehabilitation on activity limitation and impairment after stroke. *Cochrane Database of Systematic Reviews*(10).

Grefkes, C., & Fink, G. R. (2020). Recovery from stroke: current concepts and future perspectives. *Neurological research and practice, 2*(1), 17. https://doi.org/10.1186/s42466-020-00060-6

Grefkes, C., & Fink, G. R. (2020). Recovery from stroke: current concepts and future perspectives. *Neurological research and practice, 2*(1), 1-10.

Kim, W.-S., Cho, S., Ku, J., Kim, Y., Lee, K., Hwang, H.-J., & Paik, N.-J. (2020). Clinical Application of Virtual Reality for Upper Limb Motor Rehabilitation in Stroke: Review of Technologies and Clinical Evidence. *Journal of Clinical Medicine, 9*(10), 3369. https://www.mdpi.com/2077-0383/9/10/3369

Kokorelias, K. M., Lu, F. K., Santos, J. R., Xu, Y., Leung, R., & Cameron, J. I. (2020). "Caregiving is a full-time job" impacting stroke caregivers' health and well-being: A qualitative meta-synthesis. *Health & social care in the community, 28*(2), 325-340.

Koroleva, E. S., Kazakov, S. D., Tolmachev, I. V., Loonen, A. J., Ivanova, S. A., & Alifirova, V. M. (2021). Clinical evaluation of different treatment strategies for motor recovery in poststroke rehabilitation during the first 90 days. *Journal of Clinical Medicine, 10*(16), 3718.

Kuriakose, D., & Xiao, Z. (2020). Pathophysiology and Treatment of Stroke: Present Status and Future Perspectives. *International Journal of Molecular Sciences, 21*(20), 7609. https://www.mdpi.com/1422-0067/21/20/7609

Lanctôt, K. L., Lindsay, M. P., Smith, E. E., Sahlas, D. J., Foley, N., Gubitz, G., Austin, M., Ball, K., Bhogal, S., & Blake, T. (2020). Canadian stroke best practice recommendations: mood, cognition and fatigue following stroke, update 2019. *International Journal of Stroke, 15*(6), 668-688.

Liu, Y., Yin, J.-H., Lee, J.-T., Peng, G.-S., & Yang, F.-C. (2022). Early Rehabilitation after Acute Stroke: The Golden Recovery Period. *Acta Neurol. Taiwan.*

Lobo, E. H., Frølich, A., Abdelrazek, M., Rasmussen, L. J., Grundy, J., Livingston, P. M., Islam, S. M. S., & Kensing, F. (2023). Information, involvement, self-care and support—The needs of caregivers of people with stroke: A grounded theory approach. *Plos one, 18*(1), e0281198.

Lwi, S. J., Herron, T. J., Curran, B. C., Ivanova, M. V., Schendel, K., Dronkers, N. F., & Baldo, J. V. (2021). Auditory comprehension deficits in post-stroke aphasia: Neurologic and demographic correlates of outcome and recovery. *Frontiers in neurology, 12*, 680248.

Magwood, G. S., Nichols, M., Jenkins, C., Logan, A., Qanungo, S., Zigbuo-Wenzler, E., & Ellis, C., Jr. (2020). Community-Based Interventions for Stroke Provided by Nurses and Community Health Workers: A Review of the Literature. *Journal of Neuroscience Nursing, 52*(4). https://journals.lww.com/jnnonline/fulltext/2020/08000/community_based_interventions_for_stroke_provided.4.aspx

Marzola, P., Melzer, T., Pavesi, E., Gil-Mohapel, J., & Brocardo, P. S. (2023). Exploring the Role of Neuroplasticity in Development, Aging, and Neurodegeneration. *Brain Sciences, 13*(12).

McGlinchey, M. A.-O., James, J., McKevitt, C., Douiri, A., & Sackley, C. (2020). The effect of rehabilitation interventions on physical function and immobility-related complications in severe stroke: a systematic review. (2044-6055 (Electronic)).

Murphy, S. J. X., & Werring, D. J. (2020). Stroke: causes and clinical features. *Medicine, 48*(9), 561-566. https://doi.org/https://doi.org/10.1016/j.mpmed.2020.06.002

Muscaritoli, M. (2021). The impact of nutrients on mental health and well-being: insights from the literature. *Frontiers in nutrition*, 97.

Nizamis, K., Athanasiou, A., Almpani, S., Dimitrousis, C., & Astaras, A. (2021). Converging Robotic Technologies in Targeted Neural Rehabilitation: A Review of Emerging Solutions and Challenges. *Sensors, 21*(6), 2084. https://www.mdpi.com/1424-8220/21/6/2084

Orellana-Urzúa, S., Rojas, I., Líbano, L., & Rodrigo, R. (2020). Pathophysiology of Ischemic Stroke: Role of Oxidative Stress. *Current Pharmaceutical Design, 26*(34), 4246-4260. https://doi.org/10.2174/1381612826666200708133912

Premilovac, D., & Sutherland, B. A. (2023). Acute and long-term changes in blood flow after ischemic stroke: challenges and opportunities. *Neural Regeneration Research, 18*(4), 799.

Purohit, R., Wang, S., Dusane, S., & Bhatt, T. (2023). Age-related differences in reactive balance control and fall-risk in people with chronic stroke. *Gait & Posture, 102,* 186-192. https://doi.org/https://doi.org/10.1016/j.gaitpost.2023.03.011

Rahman, M. S., Peng, W., Adams, J., & Sibbritt, D. (2023). The use of self-management strategies for stroke rehabilitation: a scoping review. *Topics in Stroke Rehabilitation, 30*(6), 552-567. https://doi.org/10.1080/10749357.2022.2127651

Richards, L. G., & Cramer, S. C. (2023). Therapies Targeting Stroke Recovery. *Stroke, 54*(1), 265-269. https://doi.org/10.1161/STROKEAHA.122.041729

Robles, C. M., Anderson, B., Dukclow, S. P., & Striemer, C. L. (2023). Assessment and recovery of visually guided reaching deficits following cerebellar stroke. *Neuropsychologia, 188,* 108662. https://doi.org/https://doi.org/10.1016/j.neuropsychologia.2023.108662

Smith, F. E., Jones, C., Gracey, F., Mullis, R., Coulson, N. S., & De Simoni, A. (2021). Emotional adjustment post-stroke: A qualitative study of an online stroke community. *Neuropsychological Rehabilitation, 31*(3), 414-431. https://doi.org/10.1080/09602011.2019.1702561

Stubberud, J., Løvstad, M., Solbakk, A.-K., Schanke, A.-K., & Tornås, S. (2020). Emotional regulation following acquired brain injury: Associations with executive functioning in daily life and symptoms of anxiety and depression. *Frontiers in neurology, 11,* 1011.

Stulberg, E. L., Sachdev, P. S., Murray, A. M., Cramer, S. C., Sorond, F. A., Lakshminarayan, K., & Sabayan, B. (2023). Post-Stroke Brain Health Monitoring and Optimization: A Narrative Review. *Journal of Clinical Medicine, 12*(23).

Su, F., & Xu, W. (2020). Enhancing brain plasticity to promote stroke recovery. *Frontiers in neurology, 11,* 554089.

Swaffield, E., Cheung, L., Khalili, A., Lund, E., Boileau, M., Chechlacz, D., Musselman, K. E., & Gauthier, C. (2022). Perspectives of people living with a spinal cord injury on activity-based therapy. *Disability and Rehabilitation, 44*(14), 3632-3640. https://doi.org/10.1080/09638288.2021.1878293

Szczepańska-Gieracha, J., & Mazurek, J. (2020). The role of self-efficacy in the recovery process of stroke survivors. *Psychology Research and Behavior Management,* 897-906.

Teasell, R., Salbach, N. M., Foley, N., Mountain, A., Cameron, J. I., Jong, A. d., Acerra, N. E., Bastasi, D., Carter, S. L., Fung, J., Halabi, M.-L., Iruthayarajah, J., Harris, J., Kim, E., Noland, A., Pooyania, S., Rochette, A., Stack, B. D.,

Symcox, E., . . . Lindsay, M. P. (2020). Canadian Stroke Best Practice Recommendations: Rehabilitation, Recovery, and Community Participation following Stroke. Part One: Rehabilitation and Recovery Following Stroke; 6th Edition Update 2019. *International Journal of Stroke*, *15*(7), 763-788. https://doi.org/10.1177/1747493019897843

Wang, D., Xiang, J., He, Y., Yuan, M., Dong, L., Ye, Z., & Mao, W. (2022). The mechanism and clinical application of constraint-induced movement therapy in stroke rehabilitation. *Frontiers in Behavioral Neuroscience*, *16*, 828599.

Xing, Y., & Bai, Y. (2020). A Review of Exercise-Induced Neuroplasticity in Ischemic Stroke: Pathology and Mechanisms. *Molecular Neurobiology*, *57*(10), 4218-4231. https://doi.org/10.1007/s12035-020-02021-1

Ye, F., Garton, H. J. L., Hua, Y., Keep, R. F., & Xi, G. (2021). The Role of Thrombin in Brain Injury After Hemorrhagic and Ischemic Stroke. *Translational Stroke Research*, *12*(3), 496-511. https://doi.org/10.1007/s12975-020-00855-4

Yochelson, M. R., DennisonSr, A. C., & Kolarova, A. L. (2021). 44 - Stroke Rehabilitation. In D. X. Cifu (Ed.), *Braddom's Physical Medicine and Rehabilitation (Sixth Edition)* (pp. 954-971.e953). Elsevier. https://doi.org/https://doi.org/10.1016/B978-0-323-62539-5.00044-8

Yu, H.-x., Wang, Z.-x., Liu, C.-b., Dai, P., Lan, Y., & Xu, G.-q. (2021). Effect of Cognitive Function on Balance and Posture Control after Stroke. *Neural Plasticity*, *2021*, 6636999. https://doi.org/10.1155/2021/6636999

Zielińska-Nowak, E., Cichon, N., Saluk-Bijak, J., Bijak, M., & Miller, E. (2021). Nutritional Supplements and Neuroprotective Diets and Their Potential Clinical Significance in Post-Stroke Rehabilitation. *Nutrients*, *13*(8), 2704. https://www.mdpi.com/2072-6643/13/8/2704

Zotey, V., Andhale, A., Shegekar, T., & Juganavar, A. (2023). Adaptive Neuroplasticity in Brain Injury Recovery: Strategies and Insights. *Cureus*, *15*(9).

www.ingramcontent.com/pod-product-compliance
Lightning Source LLC
Chambersburg PA
CBHW050836260726
48660CB00006B/2273